# THE WAS SCEPTRE

Protein Sheik Fountain of Youth

Chase Duquesnay Enqi Real

**Amazon**

*the Kemetic Scientists of many thousands of years ago,  that pioneered the science we have today.*

# CONTENTS

# INTRODUCTION

I had no idea that Janurary the 20th would become such a epic day in my life. It's my ptathers birthday but also mine as a Royal Arch Mason. Janurary 20th 2019.

The reason thats important is because it was how I made the discovery that the Was Sceptre was indeed the Aorta. My first step was in discovering that the Aorta was the Holy Royal Arch in 2021. That discovery I would say took my entire life study of esoteric and anatomical study. From there it was only a few months and gallons of caffeine infused Bleu Magick until I saw it. I just saw it! I said "Is that the...."

I immediately began to  pull all the stories about the Was Scepter I could find. I had been teaching about the Ogdoad for many years without noticing the were all carrying this staff! Understanding Freemasonry as Biochemistry served as a fertile soil for many divine seeds...

It only took me a couple years to write and release the first rough draft in early 2023, called the Most High Naga. This was a very rough draft of what would become L'Goat Book Feburary 2024.

Since these discoveries it has been like trying to keep a claim to a gold mine in the Wild Wild West. I just thank God for his blessings, that I have been so blessed to be able to share. I also thank God for my father who insisted I read plenty Louis Lamour books to prep me for the Wild Wild West.

In hindsight I guess this process of understanding Kemetic Science began with my discovery that the Ogdoad or Kemenu referred the Histones. This came decades ago... I made a formula called Historic for a friend of mine who won the Super Bowl with the Giants (Jaquan Williams), he had a concussion and called me the summer before Will Smith released his movie. He had heard a bunch of my lectures on the Ogdoad and Histones and wanted to know if I could help him...

I can't wait to see what we do next. It's almost like everytime I sit down to study I am blessed. There are so many people that look to steal from me I have gotten into the pratice now of releasing a book before each insight, it slows down my ability to teach but helps with the bandits and claim jumpers lmao... Thanks Dad!

# ROYAL ARCH GENESIS

**Embryology, Aortic Arch**

Ryan D. Rosen; Bruno Bordoni.

Author Information and Affiliations

Last Update: March 6, 2023.

EXPLAINED AND MADE PLAIN BY DR. ENQI

The thoracic aorta (aorta inside the thorax meaning aorta inside the chest) subdivides into three sections, the ascending aorta,

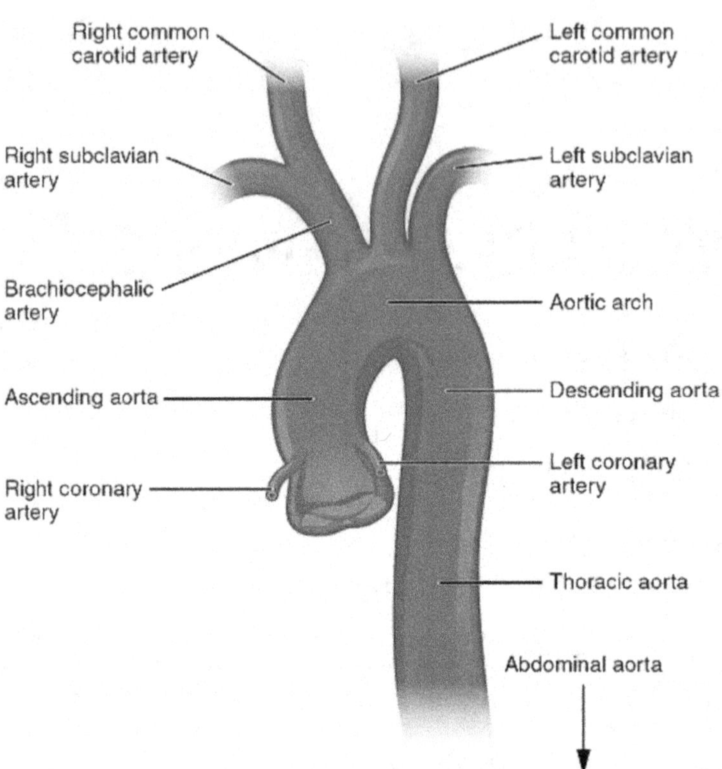


the aortic arch, and the descending aorta. The ascending (RISING) thoracic aorta arises from the left ventricle of the heart, anterior to the pulmonary artery, and rises to approximately the level of the fourth **thoracic vertebra**. The aorta then begins to travel **posteriorly** and to the left, where it is known as the arch of the aorta. The normal arch of the aorta gives off **three** vessels. The brachiocephalic (pertaining to the arm and the head) trunk, also known as the innominate (means nameless, not named or anonymous) artery, is the first branch, bifurcating (dividing in two) into the right subclavian (inserted into or under the clavicle, bones in front the neck) and right common carotid (heart to head) artery. The brachiocephalic trunk is then followed

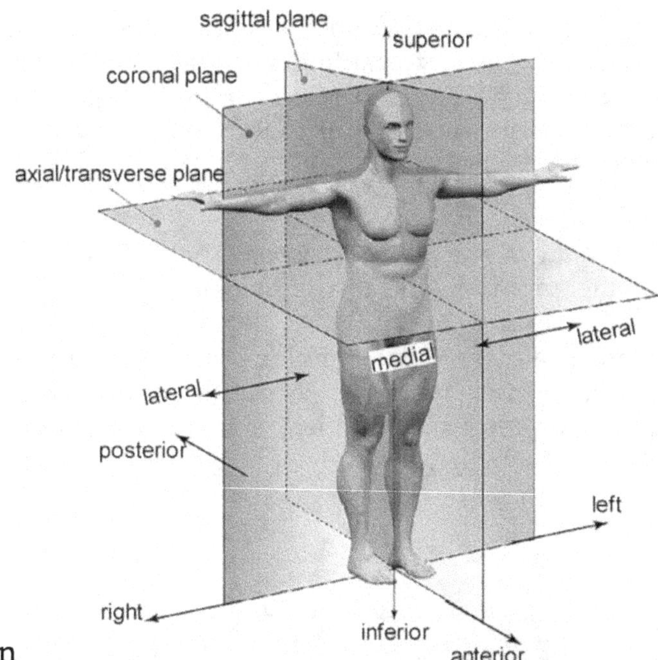


by the left common carotid and subclavian arteries. The 'typical' pattern of aortic arch vessels **occurs in approximately 70% of the population** (30% OF PEOPLE HAVE A DIFFERENT AORTA STRUCTURE). Around the vertebral level of T4, the aorta continues as the descending (GOING DOWN) thoracic aorta until it reaches the diaphragm.

## Development of the Thoracic Aorta

The ascending aorta develops as a component of the primitive heart tube. (The primitive heart tube is composed of **three layers**, which are analogous to the adult human heart. The endocardium (cardium - a combining form occurring in compounds that denote tissue or organs associated with the heart) forms the endothelial lining of the embryonic heart. The myocardium forms the muscular bulk of the embryonic heart while the visceral pericardium forms the embryonic heart tube's external surface.)

The primitive heart develops from five dilations (dilations - of enlarging, expanding, or widening) : the truncus arteriosus, conus cordis, primitive ventricle, primitive atrium, and the sinus venosus. The truncus arteriosus forms the basis for developing the ascending aorta and pulmonary trunk, beginning during the fifth week of development. The truncus starts as a single outflow tract from the right and left ventricles but is eventually divided by the aorticopulmonary (AORTICOPULMONARY - JOINING THE AORTA TO THE PULMONARY ARTERY) septum into separate vascular outflow channels. The truncal and conal ridges are invaded by **neural crest cells (NEURONS & MELANOCYTES)**, leading to **spiraling** that forms the aorticopulmonary septum.[3]

The arch of the aorta develops from multiple structures. The portion of the arch proximal to the brachiocephalic trunk arises directly from the aortic sac. The medial area of the arch, between the brachiocephalic trunk and the left common carotid artery, arises from the left fourth aortic arch. The portion of the arch distal (away from the center or geological activity) to the left common carotid artery arises from the dorsal (near the back or on the back of) aorta.

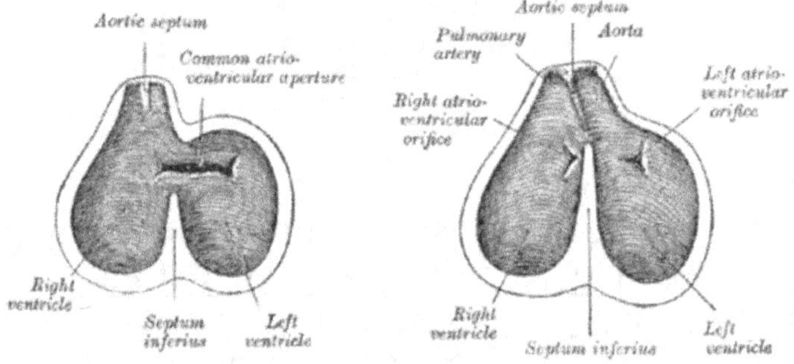


The descending aorta arises from the dorsal aorta. Early in development, paired right and left dorsal aortae are confluent (running with or fluent with) with the aortic sac. The right and left dorsal aortae later fuse along vertebral levels T4 to L4, forming a single, continuous dorsal aorta. The dorsal aorta ultimately gives off many vital branches, including intersegmental (between segments), splanchnic (pertaining to the viscera meaning tissue of the internal organs) or visceral, and umbilical arteries.[4] The dorsal aorta in this region is later referred to as the descending thoracic and abdominal aorta.

(THE ENTIRE SYSTEM VESSELS, ALL 60,000 MILES, GROWS OUT OF THE AORTA & THE AORTA GROWS OUT OF THE HEART. the history of Ponce de Leon's search for the Fountain of Youth the history of Ponce de Leon's search for the Fountain of Youth was actually a Taino Indian legend about a spring that was said to exist on the island of Bimini and a river, in what became known as Florida... calcium springs)

## The Aortic Sac

**<u>The aortic sac is the first portion of the aorta to form</u>**, appearing as a dilated structure superior (above) to the truncus arteriosus. **<u>The aortic sac then develops two horns</u>**, inevitably leading to important aortic structures. The right horn gives rise to the brachiocephalic artery, while the left horn combines with the stem of the aortic sac to form the portion of the aortic arch proximal (near to or close to the center) to the brachiocephalic trunk. The aortic arches develop from the aortic sac and

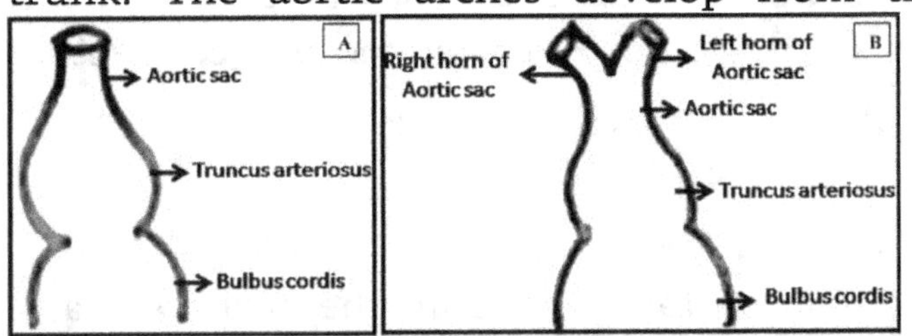


proceed to course into the pharyngeal (next to the throat) arches.

## The Aortic Arches

The aortic arches or pharyngeal arch arteries or branchial (**<u>Gills</u>** or Aortic Arches) arches develop from the aortic sac, with a pair of branches (right and left) traveling within each pharyngeal arch and ending in the dorsal aorta. Initially, the arches arise in symmetrical pairs, but after remodeling, the arches become asymmetric, and several of the arches regress. All six pairs are not present simultaneously; they develop and regress at different stages.

- First aortic arch - regresses early, but a remnant forms a portion of the maxillary artery.
- Second aortic arch - regresses early, but a remnant forms portions of the hyoid and stapedial arteries.
- Third aortic arch - contributes to the formation of the common carotid arteries bilaterally and the proximal

internal carotid arteries bilaterally.

- Fourth aortic arch - The right arch contributes to the R proximal subclavian artery. The left arch gives rise to the medial portion of the aortic arch.
- Fifth aortic arch - never forms or incompletely forms and regresses.
- Sixth aortic arch - The right and left arches separate into ventral and dorsal segments. The ventral segments are responsible for the formation of the pulmonary arteries bilaterally. The left ventral arch also contributes to the formation of the pulmonary trunk. The right dorsal arch regresses. The left dorsal arch forms the ductus arteriosus, which later closes and is termed the ligamentum (connecting tissue) arteriosum.

## The Dorsal Aorta

The right and left dorsal aortae arise from the aortic sac and receive the aortic arches bilaterally. At the level of the aortic arches, the dorsal aortae remain paired but inferior fuse inferiorly (below T4) to form the descending aorta. The dorsal aortae give off seven cervical intersegmental arteries bilaterally. The upper six contribute to developing the vertebral, superior intercostal (next to or between the ribs), and deep cervical (neck) arteries. The seventh intersegmental arteries contribute to the formation of the subclavian arteries bilaterally. The right dorsal aorta typically regresses between the origin of the seventh intersegmental artery and the site of fusion with the left dorsal aorta. The splanchnic or visceral arteries eventually give rise to ventral branches (the celiac [a vessel from the aorta entering the abdomen at the level of the T12 vertebra], superior mesenteric artery, and inferior mesenteric artery) and lateral branches (suprarenal, renal, and gonadal [ovaries or testes] arteries).

The aortic arch is made up of several layers of cells. The intimal layer consists of endothelial (The main type of cell found in the inside lining of blood vessels, lymph vessels, and the heart) cells, connective fibers under the endothelial cells, and an internal lamina.

**Endothelial Cells prove the heart & aorta creates ALL THE VESSELS!**

In the medium tunica, which is the thickest compared to the other arteries of the body, one can find smooth muscle cells and extracellular matrix. Another layer is the adventitia (COVERING OR VESSELS OR ORGANS), formed from connective tissue that wraps around the nerves (nervi vascularis) and blood vessels (vasa vasorum). This tract of the artery is essential because it must manage the blood pressure coming from the left ventricle, adapting to the speed of the flow, the direction, and the quantity of the same blood flow (mechanotransduction).

HERE IS THE ESSENCE OF THE FOUNTAIN OF YOUTH!!!

**<u>Mechanotransduction describes the ability of a cell to actively sense, integrate, and convert mechanical stimuli into biochemical signals that result in intracellular changes, such as ion concentrations, activation of signaling pathways and transcriptional regulation.</u>**

The volume of the aortic tissue is isochoric (An isochoric process is a thermodynamic process taking place <u>at constant volume</u>); it is kept constant in its form and histological characteristics in a physiological and healthy environment.

<u>On a biochemical level, blood flow generates the expression of many molecules and proteins in endothelial cells</u>. For example, the passage of blood fluids stimulates the production of a protein (proximal promoter element of 160-bp), which binds to transcription factors such as myocyte enhancer factor 2a and 2c (MEF2a, MEF2c); this path will allow the production of Krüppel-like factor 2 (KLF2), a transcription factor that protects the structure of the vessel and its function. KLF2 promotes the

production of many other molecules:

- eNOS or endothelial nitric oxide synthase
- Prostaglandins
- EDN1 or endothelin-1
- Interleukins
- Chemokines

In the development and maintenance of the structure of the aortic arch, many molecules take over. For example, in an adult structure, the passage of blood stimulates endothelial cells to express the following:

- Vascular endothelial growth factor-C or VEGF-C
- Platelet endothelial cell adhesion molecule-1 or PECAM-1
- Vascular endothelial cell cadherin or VE-cadherin
- Vascular endothelial growth factor receptor-2 or VEGFR2
- Phosphatidylinositol-3-OH kinase or PI3K
- Platelet-derived growth factor or PDGF
- Transforming growth factor-beta or TGF beta
- Endothelial nitric oxide synthase or eNOS

During development, many of these molecules play fundamental roles in recruiting cells that will build the aortic arch, such as **platelet-derived growth factor B or PDGFB**. The latter will activate the receptors on smooth muscle cells and pericytes.

Pericytes are cells present at intervals along the walls of capillaries (and post-capillary venules). In the CNS, they are important for blood vessel formation, maintenance of the blood–brain barrier, regulation of immune cell entry to the central nervous system (CNS) and control of brain blood flow.

These cells will, in turn, produce Ang-1 (angiopoietin-1), which will serve to bind these different cells together by activating the endothelial receptor Tie2.

**Vessels of the Aorta and their Embryologic Origins - Summary**

- **Brachiocephalic Trunk** - arises from the right horn of the aortic sac.
  - Right common carotid artery - arises from the right third aortic arch.
    - Right internal carotid artery- arises from the right third aortic arch.
    - Right external carotid artery - arises from the right horn of the aortic sac.
  -
  - Right subclavian artery - arises from the right fourth aortic arch proximally, the right seventh intersegmental artery distally.
-
- **Left Common Carotid Artery** - arises from the left third aortic arch.
  - Left internal carotid artery - arises from the left third aortic arch.
  - Left external carotid artery - arises from the left horn of the aortic sac.
-
- **Left Subclavian Artery** - arises entirely from the left seventh intersegmental artery.

The first classification of congenital aortic arch anomalies came from Dr. James Stewart in 1964.

**<u>There are currently no safe genetic tests to determine whether or not the aortic arch will form properly</u>**.

Now that you know a lot more about the Aorta in terms of today's Science, lets take a look at some mysteries from the past. We might be able to unravel 1 or 2. We have already unravelled the mystery of the Was Sceptre. The staff of Power or Dominion, we have uncovered to be the Aorta. This is very significant in terms of today's health, Masonic Study and Kemetic Science. Problem is the crab in a barrel syndrome that plagues us maybe just as bad as

Diabetes, maybe worse.

We fight Hate with Love, not Love of our Haters...LOL noooooo the Love we have for our Mothers and Fathers which keeps us working on advancing the culture.

Bendix Ebbell in his book The Papyrus Ebers. The Greatest Egyptian Medical Document
(1937), translated r'ib or r3'ib as 'cardia'.

In the book Ancient Egyptian Onomastica (1947) A. H. Gardiner translates r'ib or r-n-ib as opening of the Heart.

This opening of the Heart has lead to the many possible mistranslations, particularly stomach. First stomach does not fully fit contextually because there are other words for stomach. I myself took this translation on face value until I was forced to relook at the Source Material which we will review shortly!

Scholars Nunn (2006) & Hintze (1955) translate r'ib as the mouth of the Heart.

In the Ebers Papyrus #207 there is a patient whose r'ib gets "full" and the patient's face becomes pale.

#207 If you examine someone with an obstacle; his heart *(ib)*

*E :* If ₐthou examinest a man with an obstacle, whose stomach G: is anxious *("w-f)*; his face is pale,

*E :* ··*w,* whose face ·~*d,* and whose
G : his heart is beating 1; if you examine him and find

*E :* stomach makes push (hiccough ?), if thou examinest him, G: his heart *(ib)* hot and his belly raised 2. [Then you should

*E :* and thou findest his stomach hot and his belly raised (swollen ?) G: say:] This is a

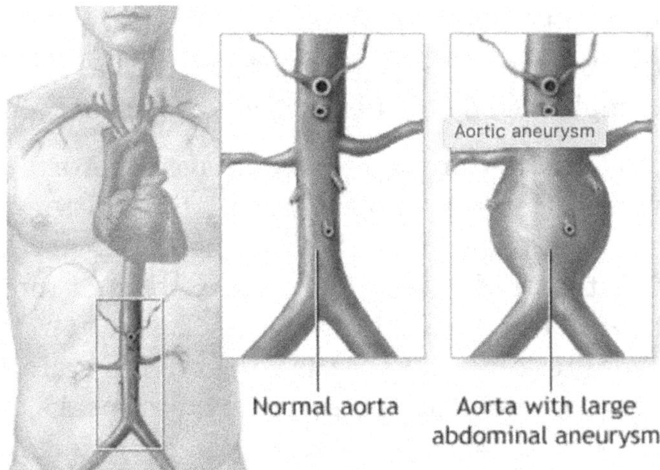



deep-seated 3 swelling

#191 & #194 If you examine someone who suffers in his stomach; he suffers in his upper arm (g5b), his breast (and specifically) in the side of his stomach 1. One says it is the w5d disease 2. You should then say: it is something that has penetrated through the mouth; it is death that draws near him

This almost certainly is a Heart Attack! Many Scholars agree, Nunn goes further to say the Green or Wadj in the reference in Cardiac Shock.

These are all supposed to be manifestations of the Stomach??? If we simply make the adjustment and translate r'ib as Aorta it will all make more sense.

The idea that these egyptologist floated, being that the Ancient Egyptians could not tell the difference between the stomach and the heart, is nonsensical to me.

There is also the mystery of why the 'ib' is not connected to the metw or mtw (H3ty, yes but IB no), the theory has been floated in these instances that the ib is sometime physical and sometime mental. In fact the IB most certainly pertains to the Mind while the R'IB pertains to the 'SideLock' of the Heart or the Aorta.

It would make more sense now that the mtw are and outgrowth of the Aorta and so they do not grow from the heart. This is further complicated by the unresolved confusion on h3ty, ib and r'ib.

Modern anatomy agrees, you have the Aorta, which becomes the vessels (mtw) and then much later still the veins which contact the Heart. The 'mtw' like the capillaries never touches the Heart. Greater still is the IB Book, please read or reread that, we explain how Arterial Pulsation drives Cerebral Spinal Fluid mechanics! This literally speaks to the vortex in the brain, that we detail in the Allergy Book. The vortex in the Brain speaks for the mind, literally and figuratively! The vortex in the brain is controlled by the Aorta! The Aorta is attached to and grows from a "opening of the Heart"!!!

# SKELETAL MUSCLE ARE ORGANS TOO...

**or·gan**

/ˈôrg(ə)n/

noun

1. 1.

   a part of an organism that is typically self-contained and has a specific vital function, such as the heart or liver in humans."the internal organs"

   part of the body

   body part

   biological structure

2. 2.

   a large musical instrument having rows of tuned pipes sounded by compressed air, and played using one or more keyboards to produce a wide range of musical effects. The pipes are generally arranged in ranks of a particular type, each controlled by a stop, and often into larger sets linked to separate keyboards.

   **<u>Mechanotransduction describes the ability of a cell to actively sense, integrate, and convert mechanical stimuli into biochemical signals that result in intracellular changes, such as ion concentrations, activation of</u>**

### **<u>signaling pathways and transcriptional regulation</u>????**

Muscular strength is inversely and independently associated with all-cause mortality, soooooo **<u>THAT MEANS IT HAS A SPECIFIC VITAL FUNCTION</u>**!

There are about 600-800 SKELETAL muscles in the human body. Smooth muscle, typically occurs AS INDIVIDUAL CELLS, meaning that you actually have billions of smooth muscles.

The human heart contains an estimated 2–3 billion cardiac muscle cells (NOT INCLUDING THE SMOOTH MUSCLE CELLS IN THE HEART), but these account for less than a third of the total cell number in the heart. The heart is composed of Neurons and Melanocytes making it a very Complex Brain!!!

THE HEART IS THE ONLY ORGAN THAT IS STILL RECOGNIZED AS A MUSCLE! The other organs have been reclassified something like this: "Although the connective tissue cells have been recognized as analogous to smooth muscle cells, they represent a defined cell population, with specific behavior and with particular relationship to the extracellular matrix".

What? This is the type of gobbledegook that never sits well with me.

Muscles have a range of functions **<u>from pumping blood</u>** and supporting movement to lifting heavy weights or giving birth.

If muscles are responsible for pumping blood and we now know that pumping blood at particular thresholds of force is a trigger for particle molecular and protein synthesis, we have the solid footing for labeling **Skeletal Muscle** as a **Vital Organ**! Our theory is, the reason there are particular proteins in younger blood, not present or present in lower amounts in "older" folks, is because the velocity of blood needed to trigger the production of these youthful proteins and molecules isn't there. In other word they lack the nutrition and/or hormesis training!

Please read or reread the Ib Book one how endothelial cells are protected! The "casts" that are formed to protect the circulatory system inhibit the max velocity which is required to trigger particular compound synthesis by the endothelial cells!

Muscles work by either contracting or relaxing to cause movement. This movement may be voluntary (meaning the movement is made consciously) or done without our conscious awareness (involuntary).

Please read or reread Melanin vs Diabetes Book 3 the Fiscal Edition.

Glucose from carbohydrates in our diet fuels our muscles. To work properly, muscle tissue also needs particular minerals, electrolytes and other dietary substances such as calcium, magnesium, potassium and sodium.

There are 29 muscles associated with the human foot: 10 originate outside the foot but cross the ankle joint to act on the foot, and 19 are intrinsic foot muscles.

The muscles of the leg are divided into three compartments: the anterior compartment, the posterior compartment and the lateral compartment. In total, there are 13 separate muscles across these three compartments.

21 muscles cross the hip to provide both triplanar movement and stability between the femur (thigh bone) and acetabulum. The word acetabulum literally means "little vinegar cup". It was the Latin word for a small vessel for serving vinegar. There are three bones of the os coxae (hip bone) that come together to form the acetabulum. Contributing a little more than two-fifths of the structure is the ischium, which provides lower and side boundaries to the acetabulum. The ilium forms the upper boundary, providing a little less than two-fifths of the structure of the acetabulum. The rest is formed by the pubis, near the midline.

THE PELVIC FLOOR IS MADE OF 14 DIFFERENT MUSCLES. The pelvis is the area of the body below the abdomen that is located between the hip bones and contains the bladder and rectum. Exercise is especially required for these muscles as we age, the control "pooping" and sexual function!

There are five muscles that form the abdominal part of the anterior trunk (home of the apron). These are the rectus abdominis, pyramidalis, external abdominal oblique, internal abdominal oblique and transversus abdominis. The first three are classified as vertical muscles and they are located near the midline. The remaining ones are flat muscles and they are located more laterally.

The back has a total of 40 muscles. There are 20 muscle pairs, one on each side of the body. Depending on how the muscles are counted (e.g. muscles that support breathing may or may not be counted), the total number may vary.

Our chest, or the pectoral region contains four muscles- the pectoralis major, pectoralis minor, serratus anterior and subclavius.

You have more than 20 neck muscles, extending from the base of your skull and jaw down to your shoulder blades and collarbone.

the face has 43 muscles

There are over 30 muscles in the hand, working together in a highly complex way.

There are 24 different muscles that make up each arm, and they control movement of the elbow, forearm, wrist, and fingers. Compared to the five muscles of the upper arm, the lower arm contains 19 different muscles that are divided into anterior (front of the arm) and posterior (back of the arm). They can be superficial (near the skin) or deep (underlying the superficial group).

How many Arteries are there in the Human Body?

1.  There are **<u>approximately</u>** 20 **<u>main</u>** arteries in the human body.
2.  Each artery is made up of **<u>muscular tissue</u>** and lined with smooth tissue, and it is divided into three layers: rigid, thicker, and **<u>more muscular tissue</u>**.
3.  There is no way to know how many actual arteries exist, the body makes new ones all the time and many are too small to count.

The arteries are also muscle tissues, the point is the next level of anatomical understanding is how 1 cell becomes so many cells and yet retains it's identity!!! The body is not so clean cut and dry! The circulatory system and the skeletal muscle system may not be as separate as we think. Remember that men with knives told us where the divisions are the body are. This is not empirical, this is the reason things change over time. Once our findings are accepted we will view the body and how to take care of the body differently!

If modern science knew everything there is to know about the heart and brain then heart and brain disease would not be the #1 and #2 causes of death.

It's only two possibilities here: A) they know exactly how the body works and have been keeping it secret to kill everyone, B) they do not know how the main systems of the body work.

Choice "a" is a non-starter because keeping the secret is suicide. This is isn't about just muslims, just jews, just christians, just blacks, just gays, just latinos, just the poor, just the uneducated, just the drug addicts... this is JUST EVERYONE!!!

There are three main groups of arteries: the systemic arteries, which carry oxygenated blood from the heart to the body's organs and tissues; the pulmonary arteries, which carry deoxygenated blood from the heart to the lungs; and the coronary arteries, which supply blood to the heart muscle itself.

Each artery is made up of three layers:

- a smooth layer on the inside
- a thick layer of muscle in the middle
- a rough layer on the outside.

How many veins are there in the Human Body?

257 VEINS IN THE HUMAN BODY? 34 MAIN VEINS

**There are literally many millions of them, especially at the microscopic and near-microscopic level. We don't give names to most of these because they're too variable from one person to another.**

Veins, unlike arteries, grow extras so there is no set number, and veins are continuous not single so they are named for the area they are in. The venous system is very large and long.

The walls of arteries are thicker than the walls of veins, with **more smooth muscle** and elastic tissue. This structure allows arteries to dilate as blood pumps through them.The veins pick up the used arterial blood which is now without oxygen. Veins do not have elastic type walls like arteries do. So, veins return the used blood **passively** to the heart where it's shunted over to the lungs for the exchange of CO2 for oxygen, then back to the heart to be pumped into the aorta under the power of whatever the blood pressure is..each time your heart beats, and distributed again throughout your body.

Veins work passively? No sir! The pressure created by the heart beat is not moving blood on the back side of 60,000 miles!

Please read and/or reread the PHD and Osiris, Diabetes & Respiration books

The largest veins in the body are the inferior and superior vena cava. The jugular vein is probably the second largest. When veins are damaged or crushed, new venous circulation develops to bypass the venous area (collateral circulation) that can no longer transport unoxygenated blood back to the heart & lungs.

The human body has three main types of veins: deep veins, superficial veins, and perforator veins.

Deep veins are located within the **muscle tissue and are responsible for the majority of blood flow**.

Superficial veins are located closer to the surface of the body and are often visible just beneath the skin.

Perforator veins connect the deep and superficial veins.

The aortic root is the portion of the aorta that is attached to the heart. Just like the nile, the top is the bottom.

A major part of the aortic root is the aortic valve, which allows blood to flow from the heart to the rest of the body when it is open and prevents blood from flowing backwards into the heart when it is closed. Like the rest of the body, the heart also needs to get blood. The left and right main coronary arteries branch off of the aortic root to provide the needed blood to the heart.

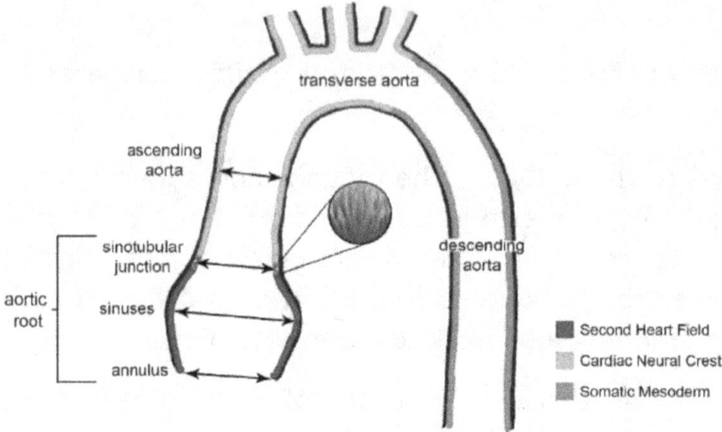


The ascending aorta begins at the sinotubular (just like a kitchen sink) junction of the aortic root and extends up and out from the heart until it connects with the aortic arch.

The Holy Arch.

The aortic arch is the portion of the aorta that is in the shape of an arch and connects the ascending aorta with the descending aorta. The major arteries that stem from the arch are: the brachiocephalic artery, the left carotid artery and the left subclavian artery. The brachiocephalic artery is responsible for carrying blood to the **right arm** and the right side of the brain, the left carotid artery provides the left side of the **brain** with blood and the left subclavian artery carries blood to the **left arm**.

The descending aorta begins at the end of the aortic arch and continues down into the abdomen. There are two parts to the descending aorta.

The thoracic aorta runs from the aortic arch to the diaphragm, which is the point of separation between the chest cavity and the abdominal cavity. It provides blood to the **muscles of the chest** wall and the **spinal cord**.

The abdominal aorta runs from the diaphragm and ends just

above the pelvis, where it divides into the iliac arteries. There are five arteries that branch from the abdominal aorta: the celiac artery, the superior mesenteric artery, the inferior mesenteric artery, the renal arteries and the iliac arteries. The celiac artery provides blood to the **stomach**, **liver** and **pancreas**; the superior mesenteric artery supplies blood to the small intestine; the inferior mesenteric artery supplies blood to the large intestine; and the renal arteries provide blood to the **kidneys** as well as the **muscles of the abdominal wall** and the lower **spinal cord**. The end of the abdominal aorta branches into the iliac arteries, which supply blood to the **legs** and the organs in the **pelvis**.

VASO VASORUM SUPPLY BLOOD TO THE BLOOD SUPPLIERS! Weight LOL…

THE HEART CONNECTS THE VEINS TO THE ARTIES AND IN THE CAPILLARIES THE ARTERIES BECOME THE VEINS!

Life is pure cell magick, Bleu Magick by our standards. The reason sitting is deadly is becomes of the message it sends to the cells and how they intern respond. Plenty of available amino acids and micro nutrition with HORMESIS TRAINING, turns the Was Sceptre into the Fountain of Youth!!!

Notch signaling pathway - Notch signaling is an evolutionarily conserved pathway in multicellular organisms that regulates cell-fate determination during development and maintains adult tissue homeostasis. The Notch pathway mediates juxtacrine cellular signaling wherein both the signal sending and receiving cells are affected through ligand-receptor crosstalk by which an array of cell fate decisions in neuronal, cardiac, immune, and endocrine development are regulated.

Thrombospondin-4 - The protein encoded by this gene belongs to the thrombospondin protein family. Thrombospondin family members are adhesive glycoproteins that mediate cell-to-cell and cell-to-matrix interactions. This protein forms a pentamer and can bind to heparin and calcium. This protein may be involved in local signaling in the developing and adult nervous system, in bone formation and fracture healing, and in osteoarthritis.

Platelet factor 4 - Platelet factor 4 (PF4) is a small cytokine belonging to the CXC chemokine family that is also known as chemokine (C-X-C motif) ligand 4 (CXCL4) . This chemokine is released from alpha-granules of activated platelets during platelet aggregation, and promotes blood coagulation by moderating the effects of heparin-like molecules. Due to these roles, it is predicted to play a role in wound repair and inflammation.[5] It is usually found in a complex with proteoglycan.

Klotho - Klotho is an enzyme that in humans is encoded by the KL gene.[5] The three subfamilies of klotho are α-klotho, β-klotho, and γ-klotho.[6] α-klotho activates FGF23, and β-klotho activates FGF19 and FGF21.[7] When the subfamily is not specified, the word "klotho" typically refers to the α-klotho subfamily, because α-klotho was discovered before the other members.[8][7]
α-klotho is highly expressed in the brain, liver and kidney.[9] β-klotho is predominantly expressed in the liver.[10][9] γ-klotho is expressed in the skin.[9]
Klotho can exist in a membrane-bound form or a (hormonal) soluble, circulating form.[11] Proteases can convert the membrane-bound form into the circulating form.[12]
The KL gene encodes a type-I single-pass transmembrane protein[7] that is related to β-glucuronidases. Reduced production of this protein has been observed in patients with chronic kidney failure (CKF), and this may be one of the factors underlying

degenerative processes (e.g., arteriosclerosis, osteoporosis, and skin atrophy) seen in CKF. Mutations within the family have been associated with ageing, bone loss and alcohol consumption.

SPARC-like protein 1 - SPARC-like protein 1 (SPARCL1 or SC1), also known as hevin (short for high endothelial venule protein), is a secreted protein with high structural similarity to SPARC.[5][6] It interacts with the extracellular matrix to create intermediate states of cell adhesion.[7] Due to its dynamic extracellular roles, being implicated in cancer metastasis and inflammation, it is considered a matricellular protein.[8][9] In humans hevin is encoded by the SPARCL1 gene.

cEBP-α complex - CCAAT/enhancer-binding protein alpha is a protein encoded by the CEBPA gene in humans.[5][6] CCAAT/enhancer-binding protein alpha is a transcription factor involved in the differentiation of certain blood cells.[7] For details on the CCAAT structural motif in gene enhancers and on CCAAT/Enhancer Binding Proteins see the specific page.

GDF11 - GDF11 is a member of the transforming growth factor beta (TGF-β) superfamily of proteins that control functions such as proliferation and differentiation in a variety of cell types. The mature proteins of GDF11 and myostatin exhibit 89% identity in their amino acid sequences, which had caused some scientists to question the regenerative capacity of GDF11 even before publication of the data from the Novartis group. The Novartis group administered GDF11 to young mice and found that muscle regeneration was impaired following muscle damage with snake venom toxin, suggesting that, much like its close relative myostatin, GDF11 has an inhibitory effect on muscle growth.

## Stanford scientists reliably predict people's age by measuring proteins in blood

Protein levels in people's blood can predict their age, a Stanford study has found. The study also found that aging isn't a smoothly continuous process.
December 5, 2019 - By Bruce Goldman

Tony Wyss-Coray is the senior author of a study that found protein levels in people's blood can predict their age.
Norbert von der Groeben

The carnival worker who tries to guess your age relies on aspects of your appearance, such as your posture and whether any wrinkles emanate from the corners of your eyes and lips. If the carny's guess is more than a few years off, you win a stuffed koala. But a team of Stanford University School of Medicine scientists doesn't need to know how you look to guess your age. Instead, it watches a kind of physiological clock: the levels of 373 proteins circulating in your blood. If the clock is off, you don't win a plush toy. But you may find out important things about your health.

"We've known for a long time that measuring certain proteins in the blood can give you information about a person's health status — lipoproteins for cardiovascular health, for example," said Tony Wyss-Coray, PhD, professor of neurology and neurological sciences, the D. H. Chen Professor II and co-director of the Stanford Alzheimer's Disease Research Center. "But it hasn't been appreciated that so many different proteins 'levels — roughly a third of all the ones we looked at — change markedly with advancing age."

Changes in the levels of numerous proteins that migrate from the body's tissues into circulating blood not only characterize, but quite possibly cause, the phenomenon of aging, Wyss-Coray said.
A paper describing the research was published Dec. 5 in Nature Medicine. Wyss-Coray is the senior author. The lead author is neurology instructor Benoit Lehallier, PhD.
'Proteins are the workhorses'

The researchers analyzed plasma — the cell-free, fluid fraction of blood — from 4,263 people ages 18-95. "Proteins are the workhorses of the body's constituent cells, and when their relative levels undergo substantial changes, it means you've changed, too," Wyss-Coray said. "Looking at thousands of them in plasma gives you a snapshot of what's going on throughout the body."
The study's results suggest that physiological aging does not simply proceed at a perfectly even pace, but rather seems to chart a more herky-jerky trajectory, with three distinct inflection points in the human life cycle. Those three points, occurring on average at ages 34, 60 and 78, stand out as distinct times when the number of different blood-borne proteins that are exhibiting noticeable changes in abundance rises to a crest. This happens because instead of simply increasing or decreasing steadily or staying the same throughout life, the levels of many proteins remain constant for a while and then at one point or another undergo sudden upward or downward shifts. These shifts tend to bunch up at three separate points in a person's life: young adulthood, late middle age and old age.

The investigators built their clock by looking at composite levels of proteins within groups of people rather than in individuals. But the resulting formula proved able to predict individuals 'ages within a range of three years most of the time. And when it didn't, there was an interesting upshot: People whose predicted age was substantially lower than their actual one turned out to be remarkably healthy for their age.

The researchers obtained their samples from two large studies. One of them, known as the LonGenity study, has assembled a registry of exceptionally long-lived Ashkenazi Jews. It was able to provide many blood samples from people as old as 95.
On measuring the levels of roughly 3,000 proteins in each individual's plasma, Wyss-Coray's team identified 1,379 proteins whose levels varied significantly with participants 'age.
Divergence

A reduced set of 373 of those proteins was sufficient for predicting participants 'ages with great accuracy, the study said. But there were cases of substantial divergence between participants' chronological and physiological age — for example, among the subjects in the LonGenity study, with their genetic proclivity toward exceptionally good health in what for most of us is advanced old age.

"We had data on hand-grip strength and cognitive function for that group of people," Wyss-Coray. "Those with stronger hand grips and better measured cognition were estimated by our plasma-protein clock to be younger than they actually were."
The study also strengthened the case that men and women, who were about equally represented in the study, age differently. Of the proteins the analysis found to change with age, 895 — nearly two-thirds — were significantly more predictive for one sex than for the other.

"The differences were striking," Wyss-Coray said. He added that this finding strongly supports the rationale for the National Institutes of Health's policy, instituted in 2016, promoting increased inclusion of women in clinical trials and the demarcating of sex as a biological variable.
Any clinical applications of the technique are a good five to 10 years off, he said. With further validation, though, it could be used not only to identify individuals who appear to be aging rapidly — and, therefore, at risk of age-linked conditions such as Alzheimer's disease or cardiovascular disease — but also to find drugs or other therapeutic interventions, like leafy green vegetables, that slow the aging process, or conversely to flash an early warning of a drug's unanticipated tendency to accelerate aging.
"Ideally, you'd want to know how virtually anything you took or did affects your physiological age," Wyss-Coray said.

While the words "373 proteins" may conjure up the image of a transfusion-sized blood extraction, a drop is all it takes for a 373-

protein readout.

In fact, a mere nine proteins were enough to do a passable job, Wyss-Coray said. "After nine or 10 proteins, adding more proteins to the clock improves its prediction accuracy only a bit more," he said. "With machine learning, you could potentially make a test with good accuracy based on just those nine proteins."

This is even more reason to study the book Osiris Diabetes & Respiration, Osiris is called "He whose windpipe is constricted". We detail in that book the relationship between having high levels of fermented fruit sugar in your blood (or as blood in the case of Osiris), with impaired ability to breath! This is going to inhibit the ability to produce the 'Growth or Youth Factors' that give us dominion of the forces of entropy (Set).

# M VS D BOOK 2
# PAGES 21-67

Melanin vs Diabets Book Two & the Gold Book are complete in terms of the What and the How! We are in a different space in this book. We are talking "plus degrees" and plus years on your life!

We have entered into the time in the world where the Body is outliving the Mind. Think about it, Ancient Egypt told us the Mind primarily extends from the Heart (in Melanin vs Diabetes Book One we explain this process), if Heart Disease is the #1 Killer…that means we are killing the Mind!

The fixes for the Heart are synthetic, they are not fixes to the main "AlgaRhythm", these fixes are superficial! The don't save the mind just prolong the life of the body in effect producing Zombies! Mindless bodies or simply mentally dead. Mentally dead people are spiritually dead people, this is the reason that Mental Illness is on the rise with drug abuse! Heart Health is Mental Health is Spiritual Health. Where the culture is and where science is today, we are going to have a F@&K-Ton of 100 year olds starting with my generation and the one behind me. The people born in the 80's and 90's are going to be very long lived but they will lose their minds midlife. Lifespans are increasing but Mindspans are regressing! The options for survival will be technology based. You will not be able to sell your SouL, you will be **PAYING THE DEVIL TO TAKE YOUR SOUL**!!! You have to do this on your own. These books have all the tools you need, but you have to use them.

1)    These books provide a form of mental workout for your Mind, separate from the information in the books.
2)    The information is the bleuprint to the future for you and your loved ones.
3)    A scientific understanding of what YOUR GOD has always intended for you, brings you close to the 1 Creator.
4)    Then the obvious things…diet, exercise, biochemistry etc…

We have covered many aspects of these discoveries thoroughly in previous texts but I think we need further Light on "Protein".

In the L'Goat book we covered Protein Synthesis and Amino Acids on many levels. Our point in this short book is the requirements and inputs for the creation of the fountain of youth. This is funny because it brings me back to the beginning of this journey with the Hair Villi. The first formula I made was Momatomix, the second Candida Cleanse and the 3rd was Hair Villi… Over the last to decades it has been upgraded into the Super Formula we know of as Purple Phaze today, back to focus this was just a little nostalgia.

Regardless to what we eat, we need enzymes to break it down the food properly. Dr. Sebi created a dangerous paradigm by stating that "Protein is imaginary or not required"! The Nano-Machines (enzymes) that we detail in L'Goat Book, are the producers of what we call Health & Wellness.

When we eat food, the small intestine is the gateway to the bloodstream, called the jejunum and the ileum. The nutrients we need are passed through the ileum, this is like a rockstar crowd surfing. The ileum has a zillion of finger-like, hairs called villi. Each villi is plugged into circuits of capillaries.

This is where the rubber meets the road, we debate food all the time but rarely discuss this process of digestion. Blood digests food and the muscles are the teeth. Did that make sense? Muscles are like distant teeth... Bad analogy... Here is some science to begin the next part of this conversation. Over the next pages you will learn one of the secrets of Momatomix regarding it's "salty" flavor! This is a key to hydration...

## Evidence of inter-organ amino-acid transport by blood cells in humans

P Felig, J Wahren, L Räf

· PMID: 4515937 PMCID: PMC433594 DOI: 10.1073/ pnas.70.6.1775

**Abstract**

To evaluate the contribution of blood cellular elements to inter-organ transport of amino acids, net exchange across the leg and splanchnic bed of 17 amino acids was determined in seven healthy postabsorptive subjects by use of both whole blood and plasma for analysis. Arterial-portal venous differences were measured in five additional subjects undergoing elective cholecystectomy. By use of whole blood, significant net release of amino acids was noted from the leg and gut, while a consistent uptake was observed by the splanchnic bed. The output of alanine from the leg and gut and the uptake of this amino acid by the splanchnic bed exceeded that of all other amino acids and accounted for 35-40% of total amino-acid exchange. Transport by way of plasma could not account for total tissue release or uptake of alanine, threonine, serine, glutamine, methionine, leucine, isoleucine, tyrosine, and citrulline. For each of these amino acids, significant tissue exchange was calculated to occur by way of the blood cellular elements, the direction of which generally paralleled the net shifts occurring in plasma. For alanine, 30% of its output from the leg and gut and 22% of its uptake by the splanchnic area occurred by way of blood cells. We conclude that the blood cellular elements, presumably erythrocytes, contribute substantially to the net flux of amino acids from muscle and gut to liver in normal postabsorptive humans. Alanine predominates in the inter-organ transfer of amino acids occurring by way of blood cells as well as plasma.

Muscle is a Organ and a Gland.

Organ - In medicine, a part of the body that is made up of cells and tissues that perform a specific function. Examples of organs include the heart, lungs, stomach, liver, kidney, skin, spleen, uterus, and ovary.

Gland - An organ that makes one or more substances, such as hormones, digestive juices, sweat, tears, saliva, or milk. Endocrine glands release the substances directly into the bloodstream. Exocrine glands release the substances into a duct or opening to the inside or outside of the body.

**Hypothesis: Musculin is a hormone secreted by skeletal muscle, the body's largest endocrine organ. Evidence for actions on the endocrine pancreas to restrain the beta-cell mass and to inhibit insulin secretion and on the hypothalamus to co-ordinate the neuroendocrine and appetite responses to exercise**

Recent studies indicate that skeletal muscle may act as an endocrine organ by secreting interleukin-6 (IL-6) into the systemic circulation. From an analysis of the actions of IL-6 and of additional literature, we postulate that skeletal muscle also secretes an unidentified hormone, which we have named Musculin (Latin: musculus = muscle), which acts on the pancreatic beta-cell to restrain the size of the (beta-cell mass and to tonically inhibit insulin secretion and biosynthesis. It is suggested that the amount of Musculin secreted is determined by, and is positively correlated with, the prevailing insulin sensitivity of skeletal muscle, thereby accounting for the hyperinsulinemia that occurs in insulin resistant disorders such as type 2 diabetes mellitus, obesity, and the polycystic ovary syndrome. In addition, it is postulated that Musculin acts on the hypothalamus (arcuate nucleus, dorsomedial hypothalamic nucleus) to co-ordinate the neuroendocrine and appetite responses to exercise. However, the possibilities that Musculin may act on additional central nervous system sites and that an additional hormone(s) may be responsible for these actions are not excluded. It is suggested that a search be made for Musculin, since analogues of such a substance may be of therapeutic benefit in the treatment of the current global diabetes and obesity epidemic.

## Skeletal muscle: an endocrine organ

Alessandra Pratesi, Francesca Tarantini, and Mauro Di Bari
Author information Copyright and License information PMC Disclaimer

Tropism and efficiency of skeletal muscle depend on the complex balance between anabolic and catabolic factors. This balance gradually deteriorates with aging, leading to an age-related decline in muscle quantity and quality, called sarcopenia: this condition plays a central role in physical and functional impairment in late life. The knowledge of the mechanisms that induce sarcopenia and the ability to prevent or counteract them, therefore, can greatly contribute to the prevention of disability and probably also mortality in the elderly. It is well known that skeletal muscle is the target of numerous hormones, but only in recent years studies have shown a role of skeletal muscle as a secretory organ of cytokines and other peptides, denominated myokines (IL6, IL8, IL15, Brain-derived neurotrophic factor, and leukaemia inhibitory factor), which have autocrine, paracrine, or endocrine actions and are deeply involved in inflammatory processes. Physical inactivity promotes an unbalance between these substances towards a pro-inflammatory status, thus favoring the vicious circle of sarcopenia, accumulation of fat – especially visceral – and development of cardiovascular diseases, type 2 diabetes mellitus, cancer, dementia and depression, according to what has been called "the diseasome of physical inactivity".

Dr. Sebi was on to something, it's a shame he didn't leave any books or students behind. He was the first that I could remember saying Iron was responsible for carrying all the rest of the nutrients. The down side is he didn't understand muscle or exercise and I think that is primarily because he was trying to build a case that "Protein did not exist"…

# 6TH SENSE

Remember the first chapter where we said…

HERE IS THE ESSENCE OF THE FOUNTAIN OF YOUTH!!!

Mechanotransduction describes the ability of a cell to actively sense, integrate, and convert mechanical stimuli into biochemical signals that result in intracellular changes, such as ion concentrations, activation of signaling pathways and transcriptional regulation. Now add on to Mechanotransduction, the fact that you have neurons and melanocytes everywhere. Your body is one big brain ran by the Heart and the Aorta is the Master Gland! Electromagnetic receptors respond to light energy. Rods and cones are examples, since they respond to photons. · Thermal receptors respond to changes in temperature. Receptors are attuned to a particular modality, but they are also more finely attuned to particular qualities within that modality.

Somatosensation is a mixed sensory category and includes all sensation received from the skin and mucous membranes, as well from as the limbs and joints. Sensory receptors are classified into five categories: mechanoreceptors, thermoreceptors, proprioceptors, nociceptor (pain receptors), and chemoreceptors.

Proprioception (/ˌprooupri.ouˈsɛpʃən, -ə-/[1][2] PROH-pree-oh-SEP-shən, -ə-) is the sense of self-movement, force, and body position. Proprioception is mediated by proprioceptors, mechanosensory neurons located within muscles, tendons, and joints. Proprioceptive signals are transmitted to the central nervous system, where they are integrated with information from other sensory systems, such as the visual system and the vestibular system, to create an overall representation of body position, movement, and acceleration.

A chemoreceptor, also known as chemosensor, is a specialized sensory receptor which transduces a chemical substance (endogenous or induced) to generate a biological signal. [1] This signal may be in the form of an action potential, if the chemoreceptor is a neuron,[2] or in the form of a neurotransmitter that can activate a nerve fiber if the chemoreceptor is a specialized cell, such as taste receptors, [3] or an internal peripheral chemoreceptor, such as the carotid bodies.[4] In physiology, a chemoreceptor detects changes in the normal environment, such as an increase in blood levels of carbon dioxide (hypercapnia) or a decrease in blood levels of oxygen (hypoxia), and transmits that information to the central nervous system which engages body responses to restore homeostasis.

A mechanoreceptor, also called mechanoceptor, is a sensory receptor that responds to mechanical pressure or distortion. Mechanoreceptors are innervated by sensory neurons that convert mechanical pressure into electrical signals that, in animals, are sent to the central nervous system. Cutaneous mechanoreceptors respond to mechanical stimuli that result from physical interaction, including pressure and vibration. They are located in the skin, like other cutaneous receptors. They are all innervated by Aβ fibers, except the mechanorecepting free nerve endings, which are innervated by Aδ fibers. Cutaneous mechanoreceptors can be categorized by what kind of sensation they perceive, by the rate of adaptation, and by morphology. Furthermore, each has a different receptive field.

A thermoreceptor is a non-specialised sense receptor, or more accurately the receptive portion of a sensory neuron, that codes absolute and relative changes in temperature, primarily within the innocuous range. In the mammalian peripheral nervous system, warmth receptors are thought to be unmyelinated C-fibres (low conduction velocity), while those responding to cold have both C-fibers and thinly myelinated A delta fibers (faster conduction velocity).[1][2] The adequate stimulus for a warm receptor is warming, which results in an increase in their action potential discharge rate. Cooling results in a decrease in warm receptor discharge rate. For cold receptors their firing rate increases during cooling and decreases during warming. Some cold receptors also respond with a brief action potential discharge to high temperatures, i.e. typically above 45 °C, and this is known as a paradoxical response to heat. The mechanism responsible for this behavior has not been determined.

A nociceptor (from Latin nocere 'to harm or hurt'; lit. 'pain receptor') is a sensory neuron that responds to damaging or potentially damaging stimuli by sending "possible threat" signals[1][2][3] to the spinal cord and the brain. The brain creates the sensation of pain to direct attention to the body part, so the threat can be mitigated; this process is called nociception. - wiki

Do you guys see where I am going with this? The 120 Day Push-Up Challenge! The Gold Book etc...

Your body has the ability to turn the amino acids you consume into a unlimited number of proteins! We don't yet have the understanding to assume we know the full potential of the Human Body. We don't even understand the Brain and Heart! If we did they would not be the #1 and #2 killers of humanity. Do not let the arrogance of the Technocrats fool you. What I am pointing out to you in this book and the IB book, is how the body routes specific information about its usage to self regulate it's own chemistry. In the L'Goat Book we detailed the process of Water as the Master Mason. In this book you are learning how the process of design works.

Need is the designer! Need though must have memory to operate from, the system we discussed in Melanin vs Diabetes Book 1 is bigger than just you! You are learning everyday not just for yourself but for Vertical and Horizontal Gene Transfer.

Vertical Gene Transfer is for all your mundane, self serving qualities. Horizontal Gene Transfer is for the species. Most people will never learn enough or acquire a skill that is required to be shared with the entire species. This is why most will fail the "Weighing of the Heart" ceremony. We are even failing at passing down strong genes vertically!

Memory is the prerequisite, it forms the basis of homeostasis. Homeostasis then serves as the purpose for building, each enzyme, peptide, protein, pigment etc... is built by Bleu Magick to facilitate Homeostasis. The mind - thought - emotion paradigm we discussed in Race Hustlers volume 5 the Movement is the crown of the system but not the entire system. The mind has limits without the body, the spirit needs the flesh to work through. The flesh must constantly be renewed.

It has been known for a long time that compound movements have much better results in terms of exercise, the reason is the internal **laboratory**. Labor-atory where labor is king and the more of the 600-800 muscles you involve, the higher thresholds you can pass. This is where the body naturally starts EPO production and many other amazing regenerating molecules and proteins.

Think about what you do with a walking staff or a cane. You put your weight on them. Pressure. Pressure is what activates the Aorta, but the right type of pressure, in consistent intervals. Diabetes is what happens when you live backwards, evil. Children are innocent, sugar immediately tells their brains to activate muscle tissue. We lose these protective mechanisms as we age or maybe we are punished for moving so much...

The legs hold up the body and are the furthest from the Heart so they are the most vulnerable to sedentary living and poor nutrition. We have 600-800 skeletal muscle but billions of individual smoothie muscle cells and remember the arteries are muscles. The Martial Artist new this thousands of years ago, Nei Dan vs Wei Dan.

Look at some basic groupings, mind you amino acids all participate together in many many thousands of varieties, but you need to consume them with purpose!

Leucine, Isoleucine, Valine - Muscle Growth

Proline, Hydroxyproline, Glycine - Collagen

Tyrosine, Phenylalanine, Tryptophan - Pigments

Histadine, Threonine, Lysine, Methionine - Neurotransmitters & Enzymes

Cysteine, Lysine, Threonine, - Immune Function

Alanine, Serine, Aspartic Acid - Biochemical Initiators

Selenocysteine - Selenocysteine has the same structure as cysteine, but with an atom of selenium taking the place of the usual sulfur. Proteins which contain a selenocysteine residue are called selenoproteins. There are over 20 selenoprotiens, many proteins that contain selenocysteine are responsible for recycling protective antioxidants such as vitamin C and coenzyme Q10.-wiki

## Potential Role of Selenium in the Treatment of Cancer and Viral Infections

Aseel O. Rataan,[1] Sean M. Geary,[1] Yousef Zakharia,[2,3] Youcef M. Rustum,[4,5,*] and Aliasger K. Salem[1,3,*]

Chiara Riganti, Academic Editor and Marialessandra Contino, Academic Editor

Author information Article notes Copyright and License information PMC Disclaimer

Abstract

Selenium has been extensively evaluated clinically as a

chemopreventive agent with variable results depending on the type and dose of selenium used. Selenium species are now being therapeutically evaluated as modulators of drug responses rather than as directly cytotoxic agents. In addition, recent data suggest an association between selenium base-line levels in blood and survival of patients with COVID-19. The major focus of this mini review was to summarize: the pathways of selenium metabolism; the results of selenium-based chemopreventive clinical trials; the potential for using selenium metabolites as therapeutic modulators of drug responses in cancer (clear-cell renal-cell carcinoma (ccRCC) in particular); and selenium usage alone or in combination with vaccines in the treatment of patients with COVID-19. Critical therapeutic targets and the potential role of different selenium species, doses, and schedules are discussed.

***Nerves and Muscles function together, in the same way that the Heart and the circulatory system are one, the Brian and the nervous system is one***. The previous sentence is so powerful it could be sold on a folded piece of paper alone as a complete book. Cheat Codes:

**Zinc** - IGF1, Muscle Building Hormones/Enzymes

**Vit D** - Hormone/Nutrient Uptake

**EFAs/Copper/Vit C** - Satellite Cells Differentiation, Myotube Formation & MyoBlast Development

**Taurine** - Muscle Cell Excitability & Stem Cell Activation

**Creatine** - Glycine & Arginine (produced in Liver/Kidney), Increase Satellite Cell Differentiation & Recycles ATP

**Chromium** - Myogenic Transcription Factor, Increase VO2 Max & Insulin Loading

**Selenoproteins (Selenium)** - Literally Build the Muscles out of Raw Nutrition & SCs

**BCAAs** - Muscle Fabric

**CoEnzyme A/L Carnitine** - Burns Fat
Water is 80% of Muscle

**Tyrosine** - Dopaminergic-Adrenergic Systems (Increased Resting Metabolism Rate, Fat Oxidation)

**Iron** - Myoglobin, Mitochondria

**Silver** - Stem Cell Activation

**Magnesium/Calcium** - Muscle Cell Signaling

**Sodium/Potassium** - Electric Potential

**Phosphorus** - ATP

**Copper** - Mitochondria, Brain/Nervous System Health

**Fucoxanthan** - Stem Cell

**Manganese** - Oxygen Boost

Keep in mind the moor we push the body the faster the Blood flows, the stronger the electric current the more DHA/O2 is consumed.

Iron/Manganese help keep O2 up, the sea veggies in Dr. EnQi's Bleu Magick help keep high DHA levels.

ATP production goes up which requires moor creatine, the lack of strength people switching from eating meat to eating plants experience is from the lack of creatine in the diet, creatine recycles ATP.

**Calcium** - Nerve Signalling

**Copper** - Ceruloplasmin, Dopamine-β-Hydroxylase, Macroglobulins, Copper/zinc Superoxide Dismutase, Cytochrome C Oxidase, Peptidylglycine A-Amidating Monooxygenase, Hephaestin and Lysyl

Oxidase & all Cuproenzymes, Copper is required for actual Nerve Cell Development

**EFA/Cholesterol** - Protection of Nerve Cells

**Chromium** - Indirect action via Sugar Regulation

**Magnesium** - Every aspect of Nerve Function

**B12/Cobalt** - Allows Metal Metabolism which is the foundation of the Nervous System, conversion of L-Methylmalonyl Coenzyme A into Succinyl Coenzyme A which is essential for formation of the Myelin Sheath

**Thymoquinone** -  Nerve conduction, Velocity, Reduced Morphological Changes and Demyelination of the Sciatic Nerve

**Vit D** - Regulates Seratonin Release/Nerve Synthesis

**Silver/Selenium/Zinc** - Protection from Bugs/Oxidative Stress

**Sodium/Potassium** - Electrical Charge

**Vit K** - Sphingolipids (Neuron/Glial Cell Membranes) & Y-Glutamyl Carboxylase (formation of VKDPs & Gas6)

**Chondrus Crispus**

Remember how we use these cheat codes, you take each one and run a search on it with your goal. These books that we write aren't designed to replace your medical doctor but to provide edutainment and teach you biochemical critical thinking. Biochemical Critical Thinking is a new term we created and coined to describe the ability to discern particular truth/fiction at a higher degree than John q pubic. In fact you will no longer be recognized as John Q Public when you speak on these subjects. You will speak, live and be recognized as apart of the 1% in intelligence quotient regarding the knowledge of the human body (KNOWLEDGE OF SELF).

Review: The blood carries sugars amino acids, glycerol, alcohols, acids, vitamins and salts. The liver must absorb and metabolize many of these chemicals and compounds.

This is the advantage that smoothies have over animal or plant based protein, more appropriately powder vs food. Food is superior to supplements in almost every way. The key to this advantage is design. The ability to tailor make your proteins. Considerations are amino acid needs, digestibility (slow digesting concentrates, fast digesting isolates, super fast digesting hydrolysates) times, specific illnesses, time of day, types of sugars, artificial colors, dollar per serving size, kidney sensitivity, water solubility, fiber content, nutrient density, …

The lymphatic system is not just a sewer system. The lymph must absorb fatty acids and nutrients as well as the blood and also functions as a system of transport. Cancer Cells in many instances travel become deadly via the Lymphatic System. This may be one of the most important reasons we have to keep the Lymph clean and electromagnetically charged!

The sugar levels rising not only stimulate insulin but inhibit the PROTEINS THAT TRANSPORT ALL OF THE NUTRIENTS THROUGH THE BLOOD! Most nutrients are ferried through the body by transport proteins, Advance Glycation End-products destroy their ability to function.

The extensions of the Aorta, the arteries in our extremities (arms, legs, the sites of amputation) run parallel to a set of deep veins. Hot Aorta blood passes cold blood returning from the feet and hands, warming the blood in these veins. This system is called a **countercurrent heat exchanger**.

Hormones circulate in the Blood Gland to Organ or Gland to Gland. Food in the digestive system, triggers enterogastrone hormones to be released.

Food increases blood flow via dilation of vessels to flood the digestive system. This reduces blood flow around other parts of the body, leading to "itis".

This increases the Heart Rate to maintain Blood Pressure, leading to blood vessel constriction.

Enter postprandial hypotension, where this process doesn't work properly, leading to nausea and/or post meal passing out. There may be underlying allergies or insensitivities that contribute to this feeling. Your body puts you to sleep to perform surgery, THE LANGUAGE OF MELANOCYTES is crucial here. The surgery is to fight inflammation and clean the blood, Blood PH is not the only thing you need to worry about. Your not using the blood and muscle appropriately. Muscle is just now beginning to be recognized as a gland or organ, BUT NOT AS WE HAVE DESCRIBE IN THIS BOOK. Muscle is a digestive organ, it is the dial, burner, incinerator for the blood. Serotonin or Melatoninn release with and post meal are based on the activity of the body, the readings of the Aorta & friends. High levels of glucose inhibits orexin which promotes wakefulness.

Eating releases enterogastrone hormones, which can increase levels of serotonin and melatonin, both of which promote sleepiness. And an excess of glucose inhibits a hormone called orexin which promotes wakefulness, Orexin works with Melanin Concentrating Hormone!

There is another set of proteins responsible for transporting nutrients from the blood into cells. The blood never leaves the circulatory system. Extracellular Fluid form a moat which another set of protein functions as transporters. This is apart of the way hormones or tissue specific nutrients reach their target. Chemical, Electrical and Geometrical differences form the basis of identification for order from chaos.

Most of these transporters are SODIUM BASED! PREFERRED RANDOM KNETICS is apart of the terminology used to describe the sodium lead binding process. Transporters can double as enzymes to catalyze the action of its payload turned substrate delivering its sodium bound 'brown box' into the cell.

In the same way as we have created the Carb Max based on your Beta Cell Activity (please read or reread Divine Mathematics & the AlgaRhythm books), your Brain & Heart activity should form your amine max number.

Carbohydrates are 4 calories per gram, Protein is 4 calories per gram, Fat is 9 calories per gram. Excess protein, becomes excess sugar, and excess ammonia based compounds (including uric acid)...

100 grams of protein is only 400 calories, 200 grams of protein is only 800 calories...

Lebron James is said to consume 30-40 grams of protein 3-5 times a day.

The Rock consumes 8,000 calories when training and  of that 350 grams (1400 calories) are protein. My point here is that the average person needs 2000-2500 calories a day, 75-150 grams of protein!

2500 - 600 = 1900 Calories left to divide amongst the fats and carbohydrates...

Walking at a brisk pace a mile in 12 minutes, burns 8 calories per minute; slow walk a mile, you'll burn 5 calories per minute.

10 Pushups burns 3 calories.

The real key is to have perpetual motion, keep moving which is why we promote 60 seconds of exercise every 60 minutes and a 20 minute walk after meals.

Basal Metabolic Rate and Resting Metabolic Rate are the true keys to Calorie Burning.

The thing I want to highlight here because we have went into immense detail on calories and exercise etc... My point here is to focus your mind on the BURNING.

## burn (v.)

early 12c., brennen, "be on fire, be consumed by fire; be inflamed with passion or desire, be ardent; destroy (something) with fire, expose to the action of fire, roast, broil, toast; burn (something) in cooking," of objects, "to shine, glitter, sparkle, glow like fire;" chiefly from Old Norse brenna "to burn, light," and also from two originally distinct Old English verbs: bærnan "to kindle" (transitive) and beornan "be on fire" (intransitive).

All these are from Proto Germanic *brennanan (causative *brannjanan), source also of Middle Dutch bernen, Dutch branden, Old High German brinnan, German brennen, Gothic -brannjan "to set on fire;" but the ultimate etymology is uncertain. Related: Burned/burnt (see -ed); burning.

Figurative use (of passions, battle, etc.) was in Old English. The meaning "be hot, radiate heat" is from late 13c. The meaning "produce a burning sensation, sting" is from late 14c. The sense of "cheat, swindle, victimize" is attested from 1650s. In late 18c, slang, burned meant "infected with venereal disease."

To burn one's bridges (behind one) "behave so as to destroy any chance of returning to a status quo" (attested by 1892 in Mark Twain), perhaps ultimately is from reckless cavalry raids in the American Civil War. Of money, to burn a hole in (one's) pocket "affect a person with a desire to spend" from 1850.

Slavic languages have historically used different and unrelated words for the transitive and intransitive senses of "set fire to"/"be on fire:" for example Polish palić/gorzeć, Russian žeč'/gorel.
also from early 12c.

## burn (n.)

c. 1300, "act or operation of burning," from Old English bryne, from the same source as burn (v.). Until mid-16c. the usual spelling was brenne. Meaning "mark or injury made by burning" is from 1520s. Slow burn is attested by 1938, in reference to U.S. movie actor Edgar Kennedy (1890-1948), who made it his

specialty.
also from c. 1300

## calorie (n.)

unit of heat in physics, 1866, from French calorie, from Latin calor (genitive caloris) "heat," from PIE *kle-os-, suffixed form of root *kele- (1) "warm."

As a unit of energy, defined as "**heat required to raise 1 gram of water 1 degree Celsius**" (the small or gram calorie), but as a measure of the energy-producing value of food, "**heat required to raise 1 kilogram of water 1 degree Celsius**" (the large calorie or kilocalorie). In part because of this confused definition, it was largely replaced 1950 in scientific use by the joule. Calorie-counting or -watching as a method of scientific weight-regulation is attested by 1908.

also from 1866

## joule (n.)

unit of electrical energy, 1882, coined in recognition of British physicist James P. Joule (1818-1889).

Heat required to change the state of water.

Water - Liquid, Solid, Gas, Plasma

Temperature is the thing that changes the state of water. Water is the Master Builder of the body's molecular machinery, tissues and Proteins!

It all comes back to water, isn't it interesting that the Aorta is shaped like a water faucet, or more correctly stated, that our creative conscious brought humans to design faucets shaped like Aortas? **Form denotes Function**.

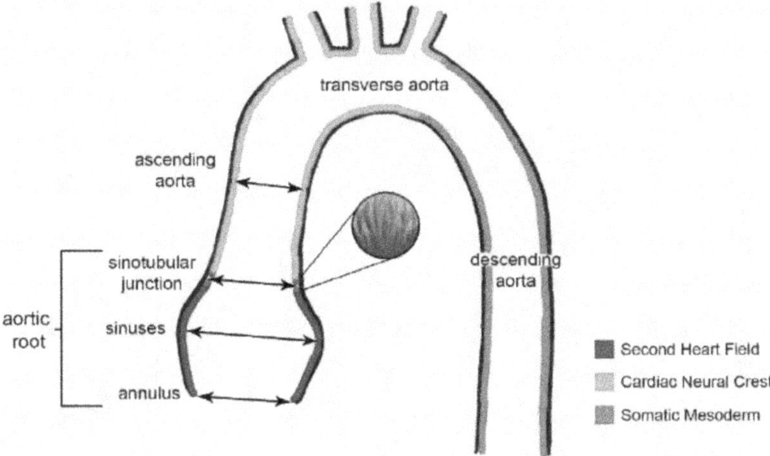


Pound for pound the most nutrient dense source of proteins on earth, is technically not on the earth, it's in the ocean! Algae. Algae is not only good for protein, it is good to protein. Algae improves the bioavailability of everything you consume it with!

Gel - proteins mixed with water.

The human body is made from Gel, by Gel. Eat & Drink GeL!

Sponsored by Bleu Magick Gel from AmericanHealer.Website

Hopefully you learn that you are the ultimate Protein Sheik!

Sheik - Family, Religious, Tribal Leader.

Your mind leads a large family of cells, in fact the number in uncountable. You are composed of trillions of cells that die and are reborn billions of times a day. In a lifetime the number of cells, with their DNA is a number so high no computer can count it. You are a God, your cells are YOUR PEOPLE. What kind of God are you, your mind is their light. Eat Right 4 Yeur Haplotype!